COMPLETE GUIDE TO LACTOSE INTOLERANCE

Comprehensive Strategies, Effective Remedies, Dietary Solutions, And Delicious Recipes For Optimal Digestive Health

DEHART HAIRSTON

DISCLAIMER

This book's content is only intended for general informative purposes. At the time of writing, the author has taken every precaution to guarantee that the material is correct and current. Nevertheless, the author disclaims all explicit and implicit representations and guarantees about the availability, appropriateness, correctness, completeness, and usefulness of the material on these pages.

Since the author is not a licensed medical practitioner, the material in this book shouldn't be interpreted as medical advice. Before making any modifications to their diet, exercise regimen, or medical treatment, readers are urged to speak with a licensed healthcare provider.

Moreover, the author has no connection to any of the businesses, organizations, or people that are discussed in this book. Any mentions of goods, services, businesses, or people are purely informative and do not indicate endorsement or suggestion.

This book's content is entirely dependent on the author's expertise, study, and comprehension of the topic. Despite having taken reasonable care to offer correct information, the author disclaims all liability for any mistakes or omissions in the material as well as for any losses, harm, or damages resulting from using the information.

It is recommended that readers use their own judgment and discretion when applying the knowledge in this book to their own situations. The use or implementation of any material in this book may result in unfavorable repercussions, directly or indirectly, for which the author assumes no liability.

By reading this book, you agree to release and hold the author harmless from any claims, losses, liabilities, costs, or expenditures resulting from or related to the use of the information you get from it.

Table of Contents

CHAPTER 1 15

Understanding Lactose Intolerance......................15

What Is Lactose Intolerance? 15

How Does Lactose Intolerance Develop? 15

Common Symptoms Of Lactose Intolerance..........16

   1. Abdominal Pain: 16

   2. Bloating:.................................16

   3. Diarrhea:.................................16

   5. Nausea:...................................17

CHAPTER 2 19

Exploring Lactose And Dairy Products...................19

What Is Lactose?..19

Sources Of Lactose In Foods.............................20

Identifying Hidden Lactose In Food Labels 21

CHAPTER 3 23

Diagnosis And Testing 23

Methods For Diagnosing Lactose Intolerance........23

Understanding Lactose Tolerance Tests 24

When To Seek Medical Advice 26

CHAPTER 4 29

Managing Lactose Intolerance Through Diet.........29

Strategies For Reducing Lactose Consumption 29

Alternative Dairy Products 31

Meal Planning Tips For Lactose Intolerance 33

CHAPTER 5 37

Cooking And Eating Out With Lactose Intolerance 37

Cooking Tips For Lactose-Free Meals 37

    1. Select lactose-free substitutes:.....................37

    3. Use non-dairy fats: 38

    5. Investigate lactose-free dishes:....................38

    6. Examine labels carefully: 39

    7. Its okay to change recipes: 39

Navigating Restaurants And Menus......................40

    1. Do your homework in advance:....................40

    2. Make a reservation: 40

    3. Talk to your server: 41

    4. Seek for lactose-free substitutes: 41

    5. Watch out for hidden lactose sources: 41

    7. Enjoy your meal:..42

Asking The Right Questions About Ingredients 43

CHAPTER 6 47

Living Well With Lactose Intolerance 47

Tips For Coping With Lactose Intolerance 47

2. Try Different Lactose-Free Products:..............47

3. Try Lactase Supplements:..............................48

4. Increase Your Lactose Intake Gradually: 48

5. Choose Dairy Alternatives: 48

6. Select Aged Cheeses: 48

7. Be Aware When Dining Out: 49

8. Maintain a Food Journal:...............................49

10. Eat in Moderation:.......................................49

Maintaining A Balanced Diet..............................50

1. Emphasize Whole Foods: 50

2. Get Enough Calcium: 50

3. Watch Your Fiber Intake:...............................51

4. Include Probiotic Foods: 51

5. Plan Balanced Meals:.....................................51

7. Speak with a certified Dietitian: 52

Finding Support And Resources..........................52

Learning Resources: 52

Support Groups: 53

Healthcare Professionals: 53

Cooking Classes and Workshops: 53

Family and Friends: 54

Keep Up: 54

CHAPTER 7 55

Understanding The Health Implications..................55

**Potential Health Risks Of Untreated Lactose
Intolerance** 55

Importance Of Calcium And Vitamin D..................56

Monitoring Nutritional Intake 58

CHAPTER 8 61

Lactose Intolerance In Children And Infants 61

Recognizing Lactose Intolerance In Children 61

Managing Lactose Intolerance In Infants...............62

Support For Parents And Caregivers 64

CHAPTER 9 67

Lactose Intolerance Myths And Facts.....................67

**Common Misconceptions About Lactose
Intolerance** 67

Dispelling Myths With Facts And Evidence 68

Clearing Up Confusion About Dairy Products 70

CHAPTER 10 73

Future Outlook And Advancements..........................73

Current Research On Lactose Intolerance 73

Potential Future Treatments And Therapies 75

Promising Trends In Lactose-Free Products..........76

CONCLUSION...79

THE END 82

ABOUT THE BOOK

"Lactose Intolerance" is an invaluable resource that clarifies a common, yet sometimes misdiagnosed, ailment that affects millions of people worldwide. Readers are given a thorough grasp of lactose intolerance in Chapter 1, including information on its genesis and typical symptoms. People are more equipped to identify and successfully manage their symptoms when they possess this fundamental understanding.

The complexities of lactose and dairy products are explored in depth in Chapter 2, which will assist readers in locating sources of lactose in food and understanding food labels to prevent hidden lactose. It is important for those who want to reduce their consumption of lactose and reduce their symptoms to comprehend these subtleties.

In Chapter 3, diagnosis and testing procedures are covered in detail, giving readers the information they need to seek prompt medical counsel and pursue appropriate medical examinations. This chapter acts as a guide for getting the right diagnosis and treatment by navigating the healthcare system.

Readers will learn useful dietary methods for lactose intolerance management in Chapter 4. This chapter offers practical advice for meal planning and dietary modifications, ranging from cutting down on lactose intake to looking into substitute dairy products.

With the help of Chapter 5's helpful advice, readers who are lactose intolerant may confidently explore restaurant menus and make well-informed decisions while cooking or eating out. People may enjoy tasty meals without sacrificing their health by learning how to cook and reading ingredient labels.

The chapter "Living Well with Lactose Intolerance," which addresses overall well-being, extends beyond food issues. By teaching readers coping mechanisms, dietary advice, and helpful resources and support locations, they encourage a proactive approach to treating their illness.

As we cover in Chapter 7, it is essential to comprehend the health consequences of untreated lactose intolerance. By providing readers with information about possible hazards and stressing the need to maintain sufficient levels of calcium and vitamin D, the necessity of proactive management is brought to light.

In Chapter 8, common misunderstandings and beliefs regarding lactose intolerance are addressed, providing readers with the evidence-based knowledge they need to make health-related choices. This chapter encourages increased knowledge and understanding by debunking myths and clarifying misunderstandings.

In Chapter 9, the book also discusses lactose intolerance in babies and children, providing advice to caregivers and parents on how to identify and treat symptoms as soon as possible. This chapter makes sure that families deal with lactose intolerance with confidence and competence by offering support and helpful guidance.

Chapter 10 concludes with a discussion of the prospects and developments for lactose intolerance research and therapy. Through learning about new treatments and current research projects, readers are encouraged to have hope and optimism for a better quality of life and management.

CHAPTER 1

Understanding Lactose Intolerance

What Is Lactose Intolerance?

The inability of the body to effectively digest lactose, a kind of sugar included in milk and dairy products, is known as lactose intolerance. This happens as a result of a lack of the enzyme lactase, which converts lactose into more easily absorbed carbohydrates by the body.

How Does Lactose Intolerance Develop?

Usually, the body generates inadequate levels of lactase, the enzyme required for lactose digestion, which leads to lactose intolerance. This insufficiency might arise gradually as a result of aging, disease, or small intestinal damage, or it can be hereditary, meaning it runs in families.

Lactose intolerance may also be transient, like when it arises after a digestive system-related disease. In other situations, it could be a chronic illness that has to be managed with dietary adjustments.

Common Symptoms Of Lactose Intolerance

Each individual will experience lactose intolerance differently, and symptoms might include:

1. Abdominal Pain: After ingesting dairy products, many people with lactose intolerance feel cramping or acute abdominal aches.

2. Bloating: Excess gas may accumulate in the digestive tract as a result of lactose intolerance, causing bloating and discomfort.

3. Diarrhea: This is another typical symptom that may happen soon after ingesting meals or drinks that contain lactose.

4. Frequent or severe flatulence may be a sign of increased gas production in the intestines.

5. Nausea: If a person is lactose intolerant, they may experience nausea or uncomfortable feelings after ingesting dairy products.

Depending on the quantity of lactose consumed and the individual's degree of sensitivity, these symptoms may vary from mild to severe and usually appear a few hours after lactose consumption.

For those who have lactose intolerance, comprehending these signs is essential to managing their illness and reducing suffering. Identifying trigger foods and implementing proper dietary modifications may help many individuals effectively control their symptoms and experience better digestive health.

CHAPTER 2

Exploring Lactose And Dairy Products

What Is Lactose?

One kind of sugar included in milk and dairy products is lactose. It is made up of two smaller sugar molecules that are joined together: galactose and glucose. All animals' milk, including human milk, naturally contains this energy-giving sugar. As the main energy source in breast milk, lactose is essential to a baby's nourishment.

Our bodies create the enzyme lactase in response to lactose consumption, which breaks down lactose into its constituent sugars for bloodstream absorption. However, a condition known as lactose intolerance occurs when an individual's levels of the enzyme lactase are low, making it difficult for them to digest lactose.

Sources Of Lactose In Foods

Although dairy products are the main source of lactose, it may also be found in certain processed foods and prescription drugs. Milk (cow, goat, and sheep's milk), yogurt, cheese, ice cream, butter, cream, and whey protein are common sources of lactose. The lactose content of these goods varies, with milk and ice cream usually having larger percentages than cheese and yogurt.

Apart from dairy products, processed foods including cereals, baked goods, salad dressings, soups, sauces, and even certain pharmaceuticals may contain lactose. It's important to carefully read food labels, particularly if you're lactose intolerant since manufacturers often utilize lactose as a filler or binding agent in these items.

Identifying Hidden Lactose In Food Labels

It's important to keep an eye out for substances that can include dairy derivatives or lactose while reading food labels. Ingredients that often include lactose include whey, curds, dry milk solids, milk, and lactose. But lactose may also go by various names, including lactoglobulin, sodium caseinate, casein, and lactalbumin.

For those who are lactose intolerant, knowing these unrecognized sources of lactose is essential to preventing pain and stomach problems. Thankfully, food producers are compelled to declare all components on product labels, which facilitates the identification of possible lactose sources.

It's important to be aware of the possibility of cross-contamination in addition to looking for components that may contain lactose, particularly at establishments that prepare both dairy and non-dairy goods. Selecting certified dairy-free or lactose-free goods will help reduce the chance of unintentional exposure to lactose since even minute quantities of lactose can cause symptoms in sensitive people.

People with lactose sensitivity may have a varied and nutrient-dense diet without jeopardizing their digestive health if they learn how to spot hidden lactose in product labels and choose appropriate substitutes.

CHAPTER 3

Diagnosis And Testing

Methods For Diagnosing Lactose Intolerance

Several techniques are used by medical practitioners to validate the diagnosis of lactose intolerance. The lactose tolerance test is one such method. In this test, a lactose-containing beverage is consumed, and the body's reaction is subsequently monitored. The hydrogen breath test is an additional technique that quantifies the quantity of hydrogen exhaled after lactose consumption. A high hydrogen content may be a sign of lactose intolerance.

In addition, the stool acidity test quantifies the level of acid excreted in the stool after lactose consumption. In the colon, undigested lactose ferments, generating lactic acid and other fatty acids that are visible in the feces. Although this approach is less popular, genetic testing may also be used to pinpoint certain genetic markers linked to lactose intolerance.

Your healthcare professional will decide which test is most suited for you depending on your symptoms, medical history, and other considerations. Each of these procedures has benefits and limits. To guarantee proper test results, it's critical to carefully follow your healthcare provider's recommendations.

Understanding Lactose Tolerance Tests

One of the main tools for diagnosing lactose intolerance is the lactose tolerance test. You will be required to drink a lactose-containing beverage during this test, usually after a period of fasting. The next step is for your healthcare professional to periodically check your blood glucose levels to see how effectively your body is breaking down lactose.

Your blood glucose levels may not increase noticeably after ingesting lactose if you are lactose intolerant, which means that your body is not able to adequately break down the lactose sugar. Nonetheless, if your blood glucose levels increase within the predicted range, it may indicate that lactose is properly digested by your body.

It's crucial to remember that lactose tolerance tests ought to be carried out under the supervision of a medical practitioner since they call for close observation and cautious interpretation of the findings. Your doctor will talk to you about the implications of the test findings and, if required, suggest dietary adjustments or other measures.

When To Seek Medical Advice

It is imperative that you see a physician for a correct diagnosis and therapy of any lactose intolerance you may have. Following the consumption of dairy products, bloating, gas, diarrhea, and stomach discomfort are some of the usual symptoms of lactose intolerance.

A healthcare provider should be consulted for a precise diagnosis since these symptoms might potentially be brought on by other underlying medical disorders. In addition to offering advice on how to manage your symptoms, your healthcare practitioner may conduct tests to establish that you are lactose intolerant.

Furthermore, you should consult a doctor right away if your symptoms are severe or persistent. If left untreated, lactose intolerance may result in various health issues including nutritional deficits.

You may get the help and direction you need to properly manage lactose intolerance and enhance your general quality of life by seeing a doctor and undertaking the necessary tests. If you are concerned about the health of your digestive system, don't be afraid to contact your healthcare professional.

CHAPTER 4

Managing Lactose Intolerance Through Diet

Strategies For Reducing Lactose Consumption

Living with lactose intolerance does not mean completely giving up dairy products. There are many tactics you may use to cut down on lactose while maintaining your enjoyment of certain dairy products.

Reintroducing dairy to your diet gradually in tiny doses is one way to find out how much lactose your body can handle. Hard cheeses like cheddar or Swiss are a good place to start since they have a lower lactose content than milk or yogurt. Dairy products that have had the enzyme lactase added to help break down lactose may also be tried as lactose-free or lactose-reduced options.

Consuming dairy products with other meals is another tactic that might help alleviate lactose intolerance symptoms by slowing down the digestive process. Try eating cheese with crackers and veggies and yogurt with granola or fruit.

Moreover, you have the choice of substituting dairy goods with lactose-free options like almond, soy, or coconut milk. These substitutes don't include lactose but provide comparable nutritional advantages. To make sure you're still receiving the necessary nutrients, be sure to choose fortified varieties that include calcium and vitamin D.

Lastly, while ingesting dairy products, think about taking supplements containing lactase enzymes. Your body lacks the enzyme lactase, which these supplements provide to help break down lactose and lessen the symptoms of lactose intolerance. Take these before dairy consumption to facilitate digestion and reduce pain.

It is possible to properly manage lactose sensitivity and yet enjoy certain dairy products by implementing these measures into your diet.

Alternative Dairy Products

Traditional dairy products may frequently cause pain and digestive problems for those who are lactose intolerant. Thankfully, a variety of tasty, lactose-free substitute dairy products are readily accessible.

Almond milk, which is a common substitute, is prepared by combining water with crushed almonds. It's a great alternative for use in cereals, smoothies, or coffee because of its creamy texture and somewhat nutty taste. In addition to being naturally low in calories and lactose, almond milk is a good choice for those who are controlling their weight or adhering to dietary restrictions.

Soy milk, which is derived from soybeans and water, is an additional popular substitute. Protein, calcium, and vitamin D are all present in soy milk, which has a nutritional profile comparable to cow's milk. It tastes somewhat sweet and has a creamy texture, which makes it a great alternative to cow's milk in dishes or drinks.

Another rich, creamy, and subtly coconut-flavored lactose-free alternative is coconut milk. It's often used in smoothies, curries, baking, and cooking. Medium-chain triglycerides (MCTs) are a kind of healthful fat that may help with digestion and offer energy. Coconut milk is dairy-free by nature.

Other options with distinct tastes and nutritional advantages include rice milk, oat milk, and hemp milk. These substitutes are ideal for those who are lactose intolerant since they are usually enhanced with vitamins and minerals to replicate the nutritional profile of cow's milk.

You may uncover delectable alternatives that satisfy your dietary requirements and save you the misery of lactose intolerance by investigating these alternative dairy products.

Meal Planning Tips For Lactose Intolerance

Living with lactose intolerance may make meal planning difficult, but with careful thought and preparation, you can make balanced, fulfilling meals that won't aggravate symptoms.

One important piece of advice is to carefully read food labels and steer clear of anything that has lactose or compounds derived from lactose. On ingredient lists, look for words like "milk," "whey," "curds," and "lactose," as they imply the presence of lactose. To decrease pain, choose dairy products that are either lactose-free or lactose-reduced.

Make an effort to include complete, unadulterated foods that are inherently lactose-free in your meal plans. Lean meats like chicken or fish, whole grains, lentils, and fresh fruits and vegetables are all great options. For those who are lactose intolerant, these foods may serve as the cornerstone of a well-balanced diet as they are full of vital nutrients.

Try modifying and creating dairy-free recipes to make your favorite foods lactose-free. For instance, swap out cow's milk in recipes for baked goods, sauces, and soups with almond or coconut milk. Additionally, you may replace dairy cheese with non-dairy substitutes like vegan cheese made from soy almonds, or nutritional yeast.

To aid in the more efficient digestion of meals containing lactose, you may want to include lactase enzyme supplements in your meal plan. To reduce symptoms and discomfort, take them before ingesting dairy products.

Lastly, remember to remain hydrated by sipping plenty of water all day long. Make sure water is part of your meal plan as it may assist with lactose intolerance symptoms and aid with digestion.

Your diet may be diverse and enjoyable while managing lactose sensitivity if you use these meal-planning guidelines and make wise food selections.

CHAPTER 5

Cooking And Eating Out With Lactose Intolerance

Cooking Tips For Lactose-Free Meals

Eliminating lactose from food does not imply compromising on taste or diversity. It creates a plethora of gastronomic opportunities! The following advice will help you prepare delicious lactose-free meals:

1. Select lactose-free substitutes: Fortunately, most grocery shops now provide a wide variety of lactose-free substitutes. Look for butter, cheese, yogurt, and milk that are lactose-free. The lactase enzyme is added to these items during production to break down lactose and make them safe for those who are lactose intolerant.

2. Try using plant-based milk in your recipes. Almond, soy, coconut, and oat milk are a few examples of plant-based milk choices that work well in place of cow's milk. They may be used in baking and cooking without sacrificing texture or flavor since they come in a range of tastes.

3. Use non-dairy fats: When cooking, consider using avocado, coconut, or olive oil in place of butter. These fats provide food with a rich, flavorful texture without having any lactose.

4. Use your imagination while preparing meals without lactose. Herbs and spices are your greatest allies for flavoring food. Try blending several ingredients to improve the flavor of your food without using dairy.

5. Investigate lactose-free dishes: There are a gazillion lactose-free recipes in cookbooks and on the internet.

You'll never run out of ideas for lactose-free cuisine, from decadent pastries prepared with coconut cream to luscious pasta meals made with dairy-free sauces.

6. Examine labels carefully: Even though a lot of packaged items seem to be lactose-free, it's important to look for any hidden sources of lactose. Make sure the product is free of ingredients such as lactose, casein, and whey before making a purchase.

7. Its okay to change recipes: You can easily convert your favorite dishes to a lactose-free version. To accommodate your dietary requirements, replace dairy components with inventive plant-based alternatives or lactose-free substitutes.

You may enjoy a broad range of tasty and fulfilling lactose-free meals without sacrificing quality or flavor by using these cooking methods.

Navigating Restaurants And Menus

Lactose intolerance may make eating out intimidating at first, but with a little preparation, you can dine out with confidence and enjoy delectable meals without having to worry about pain. The following advice may help you navigate menus and restaurants:

1. **Do your homework in advance:** Look up a restaurant's menu online and spend some time considering your options. These days, a lot of restaurants include allergy information on their websites, which makes it easier to find lactose-free choices ahead of time.

2. **Make a reservation:** Don't be afraid to give the restaurant a call if you have any questions about

the lactose content of any particular dish. Special dietary demands may generally be accommodated and information on ingredients can be obtained from the staff.

3. Talk to your server: Let them know you have lactose sensitivity when you first go into the restaurant. They may assist you in personalizing meals to meet your requirements or point you in the direction of lactose-free choices on the menu.

4. Seek for lactose-free substitutes: A lot of eateries already offer soy cheese or almond milk as lactose-free options. Asking whether these alternatives are available is not a bad idea, since they may often be changed in meals upon request.

5. Watch out for hidden lactose sources: Foods that seem to be lactose-free may contain hidden lactose sources. Creamy sauces, dressings, and soups should be avoided since they could include dairy products.

6. When in doubt, go for basic recipes that are less likely to have lactose disguised in them. You may typically safely rely on grilled meats, salads dressed with oil-based dressings, and vegetable-based foods.

7. **Enjoy your meal:** Lastly, relax and enjoy your mealtime! You may navigate restaurants with ease and enjoy tasty meals without having to worry about lactose sensitivity if you prepare ahead of time and communicate with others.

You may successfully manage your lactose allergy and enjoy a range of gourmet experiences when you eat out by using these guidelines.

Asking The Right Questions About Ingredients

Asking the correct inquiries about ingredients is crucial whether eating out or buying packaged meals to make sure they are free of lactose. The following are some important questions to remember:

1. Is there any dairy product in this dish? Make careful to find out whether any dairy products—like milk, cheese, butter, or cream—are included in the food. These substances may cause lactose intolerance symptoms even in modest doses.

2. Does this meal include any hidden sources of lactose? Casein, whey, and additions produced from lactose are examples of hidden sources of lactose that may be found in many foods. To make sure the food is lactose-free, find out exactly what ingredients were used in its preparation.

3. Is it possible to make this recipe lactose-free? Ask whether a meal can be made lactose-free if it has dairy products in it. A lot of eateries are flexible about dietary requirements and may provide changes or substitutes upon request.

4. Are there any lactose-free options? Find out whether there are any lactose-free substitutes available, including soy cheese, almond milk, or sauces without dairy. These may often be used in place of other ingredients in recipes to make them acceptable for those who are lactose intolerant.

5. Do you know of any lactose-free menu items? Ask your server to recommend dishes if you're not sure which ones are lactose-free. They are frequently able to recommend foods that are either naturally lactose-free or that are easily adaptable to meet your dietary requirements.

6. How are the components cut up and cooked? Find out how the ingredients were prepared and cooked; certain cooking methods can cause cross-contamination or the introduction of lactose. Find out how the food is seasoned, grilled, and sautéed to make sure it's lactose-free.

7. Could you tell me about the allergens in this dish? Get the dish's allergen information to find out if there are any possible lactose sources. These days, a lot of eateries provide menus or guides with a list of common allergens included in each dish.

You can make educated choices about the foods you eat and make sure they are safe and appropriate for your lactose intolerance by asking yourself these questions. To guarantee a satisfying dining experience, don't be afraid to let restaurant employees or food vendors know about your dietary requirements.

CHAPTER 6

Living Well With Lactose Intolerance

Tips For Coping With Lactose Intolerance

Although having a lactose intolerance can be difficult, you can effectively manage it with the right techniques. Here are some useful hints to get you through it:

1. Read labels and turn into a label detective. Learn about words like casein, whey, lactose, and milk that denote the presence of lactose in food. Examining labels is important because hidden lactose is present in many packaged foods.

2. **Try Different Lactose-Free Products:** Fortunately, there are many lactose-free options available, including cheese, ice cream, and milk. Try out a variety of brands and products to determine which ones best fit your tastes.

3. Try Lactase Supplements: Your body can more efficiently digest lactose with the aid of lactase enzyme supplements. To reduce symptoms, take these supplements before consuming foods or drinks that contain lactose.

4. Increase Your Lactose Intake Gradually: Some individuals with lactose intolerance discover that they can handle trace amounts of lactose without developing symptoms. To test your tolerance, gradually add foods containing lactose to your diet.

5. Choose Dairy Alternatives: Look into dairy-free options like oat milk, soy milk, almond milk, and coconut milk. These choices are abundant in vital nutrients like calcium and vitamin D, in addition to being lactose-free.

6. Select Aged Cheeses: Compared to fresh cheeses, aged cheeses such as cheddar, Swiss, and

Parmesan have lower lactose content. Moderately include these cheeses in your meals.

7. Be Aware When Dining Out: Let the staff know about any dietary restrictions you may have when you eat out. Many places may be able to fulfill your requests or offer lactose- or dairy-free menu options.

8. Maintain a Food Journal: You can identify trigger foods and make educated dietary decisions by keeping track of your eating habits and symptoms in a food journal.

9. Drink plenty of water because lactose intolerance can lead to dehydration and diarrhea. Throughout the day, sip on lots of water to stay hydrated and relieve upset stomach.

10. Eat in Moderation: Consuming large amounts of even dairy- or lactose-free food can lead to symptoms. To prevent overdoing it on lactose, control your portion sizes.

Maintaining A Balanced Diet

Keeping up a balanced diet is crucial for general health and well-being, particularly for those who have lactose intolerance. The following advice will assist you in achieving dietary balance:

1. **Emphasize Whole Foods:** Include a diet rich in whole, unprocessed foods like fruits, vegetables, whole grains, lean meats, and healthy fats. These foods are high in vital nutrients and naturally low in lactose.

2. **Get Enough Calcium:** Finding alternate sources of calcium is crucial to ensuring that you get enough of it each day, as dairy products are a major source of the mineral. Consume foods high in calcium, such as canned fish with bones, almonds, fortified plant-based milks, and leafy greens.

3. Watch Your Fiber Intake: Some people with lactose intolerance may have digestive problems after eating foods rich in fiber, such as beans and certain vegetables. To reduce pain, keep an eye on your intake of fiber and make any adjustments.

4. Include Probiotic Foods: By encouraging the development of healthy gut bacteria, probiotic foods, such as yogurt containing live and active cultures, may improve digestive health. Seek probiotic products without dairy or think about taking probiotic supplements.

5. Plan Balanced Meals: To encourage satiety and energy balance, try to incorporate a mix of healthy fats, proteins, and carbs in each meal. To make your meals engaging and fulfilling, try out several recipes and meal combos.

6. Remember the importance of vitamin D for healthy bones and the absorption of calcium.

Dairy products are often fortified with vitamin D, so if you don't get enough of it, think about eating more fortified foods or taking a supplement.

7. Speak with a certified Dietitian: If you're not sure how to manage lactose intolerance while creating a balanced diet, you might consider speaking with a certified dietitian. They may assist you in developing a meal plan that satisfies your dietary needs and tastes as well as offering tailored nutrition advice.

Finding Support And Resources

Although having a lactose allergy might often make you feel alone, you're not. To assist you on your journey, the following networks and resources are available:

Learning Resources: Acquire knowledge on lactose intolerance from credible sources, including books, websites, and medical journals. Gaining knowledge about the illness and how to treat it will enable you to take charge of your health.

Support Groups: Seek out neighborhood organizations or groups that address lactose intolerance or digestive health. These organizations could provide gatherings, learning opportunities, and tools to support you in overcoming obstacles and making connections with those going through comparable experiences.

Healthcare Professionals: If you need advice or assistance, don't be afraid to get in touch with gastroenterologists, dietitians, or primary care doctors. They may provide you with tailored guidance, suggest possible courses of action, and track your development over time.

Cooking Classes and Workshops: Take into consideration going to classes or workshops that concentrate on cooking without dairy or lactose.

Meal preparation may be made more diverse and pleasurable by picking up new culinary skills and recipes.

Family and Friends: Tell those you trust about your experience so they can support and empathize with you. Plan and prepare meals with them to create a supportive atmosphere.

Keep Up: Remain informed on the most recent findings and advancements about lactose intolerance and digestive health. Being knowledgeable may assist you in making well-informed choices about your lifestyle and food, as knowledge is power.

You may successfully manage lactose intolerance and have a happy, healthy lifestyle by putting these techniques into practice and getting help from a variety of sources.

CHAPTER 7

Understanding The Health Implications

Potential Health Risks Of Untreated Lactose Intolerance

If left untreated, lactose intolerance may cause several health problems that can negatively impact your general health. Digestion discomfort, including symptoms such as gas, bloating, diarrhea, and cramping in the stomach, is one of the main concerns. The degree of lactase insufficiency and the quantity of lactose ingested by the person might influence the severity of these symptoms.

Chronic stomach pain may also negatively affect your quality of life by making meals less enjoyable, causing social awkwardness, and sometimes making you feel embarrassed in public. In addition to short-term pain, prolonged exposure to lactose without appropriate treatment might lead to long-term issues.

Undernourishment poses a serious concern. People with lactose sensitivity may completely forego dairy products, which are important providers of vitamin D and calcium. Osteoporosis, a disorder marked by weakening bones that are more prone to fractures, is one ailment that is more likely to develop if these nutrients are not consumed in sufficient amounts.

Moreover, if lactose intolerance symptoms are ignored, the gastrointestinal system may eventually become inflamed and damaged. This may make you more vulnerable to further stomach issues or problems.

Importance Of Calcium And Vitamin D

Healthy bones and general well-being depend on calcium and vitamin D. In addition to being essential for healthy bones, calcium is also involved in hormone production, nerve transmission, and muscle contraction. In the meanwhile, vitamin D strengthens the immune system and facilitates calcium absorption.

Milk, cheese, and yogurt are dairy items that are high in calcium and vitamin D. But those who are intolerant to lactose may find it difficult to eat these meals without feeling uncomfortable. Thankfully, there are substitute sources of these nutrients, including leafy greens, fortified orange juice, almonds, tofu, and plant-based milk.

Those who are lactose intolerant must make sure they are receiving enough calcium and vitamin D via their diet or supplements. Sustaining general health, avoiding fractures, and preserving bone density all depend on getting an adequate intake of these nutrients.

Monitoring Nutritional Intake

To manage lactose intolerance and make sure you're providing your body with the nutrients it needs without aggravating symptoms, you must closely check your nutritional intake. Maintaining a food journal will help you determine which foods and drinks are lactose intolerant as well as how your body responds to them.

Make sure to include low- or no-lactose dairy substitutes in your meal preparation. Supermarkets have a large selection of dairy-free options manufactured from soy, almond, coconut, or rice, as well as lactose-free cheese, yogurt, and milk.

Furthermore, be aware that certain medicines, supplements, and processed foods may include hidden sources of lactose. You may assist yourself minimize unintentional lactose exposure while eating out by reading ingredient labels and asking questions.

In addition, supplements could be required to guarantee sufficient consumption of calcium and vitamin D, particularly in cases when food sources are scarce. See a doctor or certified nutritionist to find the right dose for you, taking into account your unique requirements.

Despite lactose sensitivity, you may reduce symptoms and maintain optimum health by proactively regulating your food intake and being aware of possible sources of lactose. You may live a happy and healthy life by keeping a close eye on your nutrition and making regular lifestyle and dietary changes.

CHAPTER 8

Lactose Intolerance In Children And Infants

Recognizing Lactose Intolerance In Children

Since the symptoms of lactose intolerance are often confused with those of other disorders, diagnosing it in youngsters may be challenging. Still, there are a few critical indicators to be aware of. Gastrointestinal distress, which includes bloating, gas, diarrhea, and stomach cramps, is one of the most typical symptoms, particularly after the use of dairy products. Children may also have trouble gaining weight, feel nauseous, or vomit.

Parents need to monitor their child's eating patterns and any negative responses they may have from eating foods high in lactose. Maintaining a meal journal might be useful in seeing trends and possible symptom causes.

Furthermore, a child's risk of developing lactose intolerance is increased if there is a family history of the condition or other dairy-related problems.

It is recommended for parents to speak with a physician or other healthcare professional if they have any suspicions that their kid may be lactose intolerant. To confirm the diagnosis, they may do tests like a stool acidity test or a hydrogen breath test. Following confirmation of lactose intolerance, parents may collaborate with medical specialists to create a treatment strategy specific to their child's requirements.

Managing Lactose Intolerance In Infants

Infants with lactose intolerance need extra attention and care since they primarily depend on milk for sustenance in their early years of life. When a newborn is diagnosed with lactose intolerance, there are a few ways to make sure they get enough nutrients without feeling uncomfortable.

Using a lactose-free formula made especially for babies who are lactose intolerant is one strategy. These easily accessible formulations are full of all the nutrients required for normal development and growth. If their infant is lactose intolerant, some parents may decide to breastfeed instead of giving them dairy items in their diet.

Parents need to be careful while introducing solid meals to their babies in addition to modifying their diet. Read food labels carefully and steer clear of anything that can aggravate symptoms since certain foods may contain hidden sources of lactose. It is possible to determine which meals are well-tolerated and which should be avoided by introducing new foods gradually and keeping an eye out for any negative responses.

A pediatrician's checkups are necessary to track the infant's development and make sure they are getting enough food. Healthcare professionals may also assist parents in overcoming the difficulties associated with controlling their infant's lactose intolerance.

Support For Parents And Caregivers

Although raising a kid with lactose intolerance may be difficult, parents and other caregivers don't have to do it alone—there are tools and support systems in place to assist. Making connections with other parents who have dealt with children's lactose intolerance in the past might provide insightful information and helpful suggestions.

For parents of kids with dietary restrictions, there is a plethora of online forums and support groups that provide a venue for inquiries, experience sharing, and getting help from others going through similar struggles. Healthcare professionals may also give advice on how to prepare meals, add nutritional supplements, and make sure the kid eats a balanced diet.

Parents must discuss their child's dietary requirements and any limitations they may have with educators, caretakers, and other family members. This may guarantee that everyone is aware of how to support the child's dietary needs and assist minimize unintentional exposure to items containing lactose.

Parents and other caregivers may successfully fulfill the requirements of children with lactose intolerance and promote their growth by creating a solid support system and being up to date on lactose intolerance management techniques.

CHAPTER 9

Lactose Intolerance Myths And Facts

Common Misconceptions About Lactose Intolerance

Many times, lactose intolerance is misinterpreted, which results in misunderstandings about the illness. A frequent misperception is that a milk allergy and lactose intolerance are the same thing. Even though they are related to dairy, they are two different conditions. A milk allergy is an immunological reaction to the proteins in milk, while lactose intolerance is caused by the body's inability to digest lactose, the sugar contained in milk.

Another myth is that those who have lactose sensitivity need to stay away from all dairy products. In actuality, lactose intolerance varies in degree, and some people may tolerate modest quantities of foods that contain lactose without developing symptoms. To assist those with lactose intolerance to enjoy dairy without discomfort, lactase enzyme supplements and lactose-free dairy products are now available.

Another myth is that people with lactose intolerance are limited to certain ethnic groups. Although, indeed, those of East Asian, African, and Native American heritage are more likely to have lactose intolerance, it may affect persons from any ethnic background.

Dispelling Myths With Facts And Evidence

It's critical to comprehend the science behind lactose intolerance to debunk these misconceptions. When the body does not produce enough of the enzyme lactase, which is required to convert lactose into simpler sugars that the body can absorb, lactose intolerance develops. Insufficient lactase causes lactose to stay undigested in the digestive tract, resulting in symptoms including gas, diarrhea, bloating, and discomfort in the abdomen.

Contrary to common assumptions, lactose intolerance is a natural variation in human physiology rather than an illness. In actuality, lactase declines to some extent with age for the majority of individuals globally, irrespective of race. The most prevalent cause of lactose intolerance is primary lactase insufficiency, which is characterized by a decrease in lactase activity.

It's also crucial to remember that each person's level of lactose intolerance varies. Some people may not show any symptoms until they've had a significant quantity of lactose, whereas others could be sensitive to even small quantities. The intensity of symptoms may also be influenced by variables such as underlying medical disorders, gastrointestinal health, and heredity.

Clearing Up Confusion About Dairy Products

Contrary to popular belief, people with lactose sensitivity cannot consume any dairy products; nevertheless, there are several low- or lactose-free choices available. Hard cheeses like Parmesan, Swiss, and cheddar have little lactose content and are usually accepted by those who are lactose intolerant. Similarly, since the bacteria aid in the breakdown of lactose, yogurt with live and active cultures may be simpler to stomach.

There are several choices available manufactured from plant-based sources, including soy, almond, coconut, and oat, for individuals who prefer milk substitutes. You may use these naturally lactose-free dairy substitutes in recipes and drinks instead of cow's milk.

To assist people with lactose intolerance digest lactose more efficiently, lactase enzyme supplements are sold over-the-counter in addition to lactose-free dairy products and milk substitutes. It is possible to avoid or lessen the severity of symptoms by taking these supplements before ingesting dairy-containing meals.

People with lactose intolerance may continue to enjoy dairy products as part of a balanced diet without experiencing discomfort if common misconceptions about the illness are dispelled and they are aware of the various management options. Seeking advice from a medical professional or certified dietitian may also provide tailored direction and assistance in properly managing lactose intolerance.

CHAPTER 10

Future Outlook And Advancements

Current Research On Lactose Intolerance

Scientists are exploring a range of topics in the field of lactose intolerance research to expand on our knowledge and enhance management approaches for those who suffer from this illness. Genetics is one important field of study. Scholars are delving into the genetic underpinnings of lactose intolerance to pinpoint certain gene variants that predispose people to this ailment. Scientists want to identify these genetic markers and create individualized lactose intolerance management strategies.

Furthermore, studies on the gut microbiota and lactose intolerance are still being conducted. The makeup of the gut flora may affect how the body breaks down lactose, and scientists are looking at methods to change the microbiome to help those with lactose intolerance. Beneficial bacteria called probiotics are being studied for their ability to help people with lactose intolerance and lessen gastrointestinal distress.

Moreover, improvements in diagnostic methods are improving our capacity to precisely diagnose lactose intolerance. More effective and easy non-invasive techniques to identify lactose intolerance are being developed by researchers. These include genetic testing and breath tests. With the use of these diagnostic technologies, medical professionals may better customize treatment regimens to each patient's unique requirements, improving patient outcomes and quality of life.

Potential Future Treatments And Therapies

Numerous possible cures and treatments for lactose intolerance are in the works as research keeps developing. Enzyme replacement therapy is one method that shows promise. People who are lactose intolerant may benefit from oral administration of lactase and other digestive enzymes to improve their ability to digest dairy products. The safety and effectiveness of this medication are being evaluated in clinical studies, which gives hope to those who are suffering from the symptoms of lactose intolerance.

Gene therapy is an additional research option. Researchers are looking at gene-editing methods that could be able to fix genetic defects linked to lactose intolerance and restore the body's capacity to make lactase. Gene therapy shows promise as a long-term treatment for those with severe types of lactose intolerance, even if it is still in the preliminary phases.

Dietary changes remain an essential part of controlling lactose intolerance, even in addition to medication therapies. Researchers are looking at novel approaches to produce dairy products that have low- or no-lactose while maintaining their nutritional value and consumer-pleasing flavors. With the help of these developments in food science, those who are lactose intolerant will have more alternatives for enjoying dairy products without feeling uncomfortable or having digestive problems.

Promising Trends In Lactose-Free Products

Due to rising consumer demand for dairy substitutes and increased knowledge of lactose intolerance, the market for lactose-free goods has been expanding significantly.

In response to consumer demand, producers have created a range of lactose-free products, such as ice cream, cheese, yogurt, and milk. These items are ideal for those with lactose intolerance since they are produced using lactase enzyme or other lactose-digesting technology to eliminate or break down lactose.

Moreover, developments in food technology have made it possible to produce plant-based dairy substitutes comprised of soy, almond, coconut, and oat flour. Lactose-intolerant people now have access to a wide range of dairy-free choices that taste and feel much like conventional dairy products thanks to these plant-based substitutes. Furthermore, plant-based dairy substitutes are equivalent to dairy in terms of nutrition since they are often enriched with vitamins and minerals.

Furthermore, a lot of food producers include lactose-free components in a variety of processed meals and drinks, thus lactose-free items are available outside of the dairy aisle. Thanks to this development, people who are lactose intolerant may now eat a variety of goods without constantly reading labels to look for hidden lactose sources.

In conclusion, there is a bright future ahead for lactose intolerance due to the continuous research that is advancing product innovation, diagnosis, and therapy. People with lactose intolerance should anticipate better management techniques and an expanding range of lactose-free choices to accommodate their dietary requirements and preferences as our knowledge of the disease continues to advance.

CONCLUSION

In summary, the inability of the body to adequately digest lactose, the sugar included in milk and dairy products, causes lactose intolerance, a common digestive condition. Lactase is an enzyme that breaks down lactose into simpler sugars for the small intestine to absorb. A lactase shortage causes this illness. Although not fatal, lactose intolerance may have a substantial negative influence on a person's quality of life by causing unpleasant symptoms including gas, bloating, diarrhea, and discomfort in the abdomen after ingesting dairy products.

Making dietary adjustments to reduce or eliminate lactose intake is part of managing lactose intolerance. This might include switching from dairy products to lactose-free ones, including soy, almond, or coconut-based dairy substitutes or lactose-free milk.

To aid in better lactose digestion, lactase-containing enzyme supplements may be given before dairy consumption.

In addition, those who are lactose intolerant must read food labels carefully and be aware of potential hidden sources of lactose in processed foods and prescription drugs. Since dairy products are the main source of calcium and vitamin D, it is essential to maintain a balanced diet rich in these minerals to avoid shortages. To assist satisfy nutritional demands, foods and drinks fortified with calcium as well as calcium supplements may be included.

Those exhibiting lactose intolerance symptoms must speak with a medical practitioner for a precise diagnosis and individualized treatment plan. Even while dietary changes might help manage lactose intolerance, it's important to rule out any underlying diseases that may be causing similar symptoms.

All things considered, people with lactose intolerance may successfully manage their illness and have pleasant, symptom-free lives with the right knowledge, dietary modifications, and medical advice.

THE END